TABLE OF CONTENTS

The Headache Pain Cure

The Arthritis Pain Cure

The Headache Pain Cure

How To Find Headache Pain Relief And Live A Happy Pain Free Life!

By

Michele Gilbert

<u>Visit My Amazon Author Page</u>

Dedicated to those who choose to stretch beyond their own limits and to seek a more abundant and fulfilling life.

Your thoughts are creative.

Michele Gilbert

My Free Gift To You!

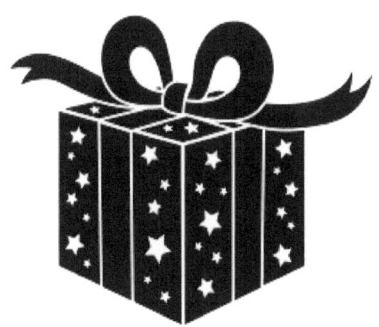

As a way of saying thank you for downloading my book, I am willing to give you access to a selected group of readers who (every week or so) receive inspiring, life-changing kindle books at deep discounts, and sometimes even absolutely free.

Wouldn't it be great to get amazing Kindle offers delivered directly to your inbox?

Wouldn't it be great to be the first to know when I'm releasing new fresh and above all sharply discounted content?

But why would I do something like this?

Why would I offer my books at such a low price and even give them away for free when they took me countless hours to produce?

Simple…. Because I Want To Spread The Word.!

For a few short days Amazon allows Kindle authors to promote their newly released books by offering them deeply discounted (up to 70% price discounts and even for free. This allows us to spread the word extremely quickly allowing users to download thousands and thousands of copies in a very short period of time.

Once the timeframe has passed, these books will revert back to their normal selling price. That's why you will benefit from being the first to know when they can be downloaded for free!

So are you ready to claim your weekly Kindle books?

You are just one click away! Follow the link below and sign up to start receiving awesome content

Thank you and Enjoy!

Introduction

I want to thank you and congratulate you for downloading the book, *"The Headache Pain Cure: How to Find Headache Pain Relief and Live a Happy Pain Free Life!"* This book contains proven steps and strategies on how to relieve the pain provoked by different types of headaches.

In this book we are offering detailed explanations on different causes and types of headaches and different approaches in treating the problem. We have offered some proven steps in relieving pain, but also preventing it from happening. Remember it is always better to try to prevent it than to cure it. If you have developed a chronic headache problem, this book will help you learn comprehensive ways in addressing your health problem and maintaining a healthy and active life.

Thanks again for downloading this book, I hope you enjoy it!

What are the causes and symptoms of headaches?

The head is one of the most common aching parts of the body. There are different types of headaches but one thing is sure, they are one of the most limiting types of soreness because they can block our everyday activities and duties. Because this condition is so widely spread doctors have constructed a classification for the types of headaches that help them address and treat the problem. The most types of headaches can be classified in three subcategories, primary, secondary and cranial neuralgias following by facial pain and other types of condition. Under these subcategories there are also different types of pain, so the primary headaches are differentiated into tension, migraine and cluster, in which the tension headaches are the most common type of the condition and are treated by over-the-counter medications for which a prescription is not needed. Tension headaches occur more frequently among women then man. 1 in 20 people in the world suffer from this type of the condition. Migraine headaches are the second typical form of the headaches. They affect children, as well as adults. Before puberty both sexes are affected equally, but after this period women are more likely to suffer from migraines. Primary headaches do affect significantly on the quality of the lifestyle. Secondary headaches represent a symptom on an injury or underlying illness so you should be careful about them. The structural problems range from infected teeth or sinus to meningitis or internal bleeding. If you experience headaches you should consult your doctor to be sure that there is not some deeper rooted reason of your health condition. There are some following symptoms that indicate the seriousness of the condition, so if you feel these sensations, you should contact your doctor immediately. These symptoms are: fever, stiff neck, and change in behavior, vomiting or weakness.

Headache is defined as a pain arising from the head or upper part of the neck. The pain is generated from the tissues surrounding the brain, because the brain is not neurologically structured to cause the sensation of pain, meaning that it has no nerves that give rise to the sensation of pain. The periosteum that surrounds bones; muscles surrounding the skull, sinuses, eyes, and ears; and meninges that cover the surface of the brain and spinal cord, arteries, veins, and nerves can become inflamed and cause a headache. There are different types of pain, ranging from dull constant sensation to sharp intense pain.

Tension headaches

Because the tension type of headache is most wide spread you will now learn what the symptoms of the condition are and get more detailed information about it. Common presentation of tension headaches are pain that begins in the back of the head and upper neck and includes the sensation of pressure, the most intense pressure is felt above the eyebrows. The pain can vary in intensity but it is usually not disabling, it does not prevent you for doing your day to day activities. The pain is not followed by any other bodily sensations as vomiting or audio/visual sensitivity. The appearance of the pain is sporadic and it is usually not frequent.

The causes of this type of headache are unknown. It is commonly thought, among the professionals, that the pain is caused by a contraction of muscles surrounding the skull. This type of headaches can occur due to the physical or emotional stress. Physical stress is caused by a hard and long term labor, or a job that requires long sitting hours, especially when the working on the computer is included.

If you think that you may suffer from tension headaches you should visit your doctor. The diagnosis is made by your health history. The person who is diagnosed with this condition usually complaints about mild or moderate aches, located on both sides of the head. Tension headache sufferers do not notice the worsening of the pain with the increase of the activity. Still, even though tension headaches are not life threatening, daily activities could become more difficult to accomplish.

Drug treatment of headaches

In this book you will learn the ways in treating the primary type of headaches, mostly tension headaches. As we have mentioned, some over the counter drugs are most commonly used in relieving the tension headache pain, such as aspirin, ibuprofen, acetaminophen and naproxen. When using these drugs you should keep some things in mind. Aspirin should not be used in children younger than 14 years of age, because this drug can be a trigger in developing Reye's syndrome, a life threatening neurological condition. People are usually not careful with this drug because it is most common used in different type of conditions and for different aches to be relieved. There are some serious side effects that can occur when using the drug, such as gastrointestinal bleeding, heartburn, ulcers and anaphylaxis, a life threatening allergic reaction. Ibuprofen is known for the possibility of causing gastrointestinal bleeding, nausea, rash, liver damage and gastrointestinal upset. Acetaminophen seems as the least harmful of the commonly used drugs. There is still risk of developing changes in blood and liver damage. Naproxen is known for having similar side effects as ibuprofen, including vomiting, rash and liver damage. There are also some other pain relievers that are prescribed if the person is experiencing headache, such as fenoprofen, flubiprofen, nabumetone etc. These pain relief meds are usually safe when used as directed, but, besides the side effects you should keep these facts in mind.

- Get informed about the active ingredients in every medicine to be sure if you are allowed to use the meds. Maybe you are allergic to some ingredient. Read the label thoroughly and carefully.
- Never exceed the recommended dosage on the package
- Take care of the way you are using this type of drugs, it is easy to over-medicate yourself.
- You should ask your doctor for approval before using the meds that contain aspirin, ibuprofen or naproxen, especially if you have a bleeding problem, asthma, if you have underwent any type of surgery recently or you are about to have one. You should also ask for advice if you have ulcers, any type of kidney or liver disorder.

When using pain relief drugs avoid excessive caffeine usage and mixing it with other over-the-counter meds. Any medication containing barbiturates or narcotics should be used sparingly. If you notice that you are using the meds more than twice a week, you should visit a doctor who will prescribe you a headache therapy. Overuse of symptomatic pain relief drugs can cause more frequent headaches and resistance to the medication.

Biofeedback therapy

There are some automatic functions in our body that occur without us being aware of them. Breathing is the best example of these processes and functions, because we are not aware that we are breathing, we do it naturally without thinking about it. Biofeedback is a way of gaining control over these processes in order to achieve a more relaxed state of your organism. You will learn more about your automatic bodily activities, which will help you in controlling the functions of your body and also in relieving the pain. Biofeedback is a practice that involves learning how your body functions and learning how to control it.

There are different types of biofeedback therapy. EMG biofeedback is based on the muscle tension control, while on the other hand thermal biofeedback and blood flow feedback relate to the information regarding blood flow. Never mind which type of biofeedback therapy you choose it will all begin the same way. Individual is hooked up to a computer that shows the physiology of one's body. According to specialist thermal biofeedback is the most effective in treating the headaches. A person suffering from headaches will learn how to monitor the severity of the pain, or even prevent it, if using the therapy 20-30 minutes, 2-3 times a week.

Biofeedback therapy is especially effective when combined with relaxation techniques. These techniques are based to teach you how to achieve a physical and mental state of calm and relaxation. You sure do have some activities that you find relaxing, but, relaxation techniques are actually a systematic set of activities that you have to learn in order to apply them right. Relaxation procedures are crucial in curing primary type of headaches, because, as we have mentioned, they are in most cases caused by a stressful everyday life. Relaxation training and techniques slow down the sympathetic nervous system which is responsible for stress response.

There are different relaxation techniques that you can use for achieving your emotional and physical balance. One of which is the deep breathing technique. You should place one hand on your chest and one on your abdomen to be aware of the breathing process. Afterwards you should breathe in through your nose and exhale through the mouth, very slowly. Whilst breathing try to pull your breath towards your belly, and feel it filling with air. This process you will have to practice to get the best results. But once you have learned it, it will help you to maintain the emotional calm, much needed for avoiding stress that can trigger your headaches. Besides deep breathing there are progressive muscle relaxation and many different relaxation techniques, that you can be thought by a professional if you want to try them out. Remember, it is always better to avoid chemical treatment in favor of alternative ways of relieving pain. A stress and pain free life is what you want to achieve, and this could be done by a regular practice and techniques that would do you good.

Exercises that will relieve your pain

Besides the generally healthy way of life, enough sleep, avoiding stress etc., there are some exercises that could help you prevent headaches. These exercises take 15-20 minutes a day, but are effective in reducing the risk of developing headache condition and attacks of pain. **Gentle neck and shoulder exercises may be used to relax and stretch strained, shortened muscles.** This can reduce tension and decrease the risk of headaches triggered by muscle tension. These exercises that you will now have a chance to learn are equally effective for tension headache sufferers and migraine sufferers.

- **Neck rotation** - Rotate your head till you look straight out over one shoulder, all the way keeping your head in the same level. When you reach the point, stay in this position for 10-20 minutes, and look down at your shoulder. Return your head to a starting position, and do the same other way around.

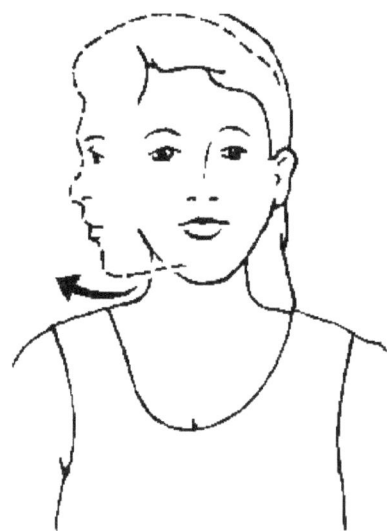

- **Neck retraction** - Squeeze your shoulder blades together and whilst in this position pull your head straight back, keeping in mind to keep it level. Stay in this position for 10 seconds and get to the starting position. Repeat this movement 10 times. Remember do it slowly, you should not feel any pain.

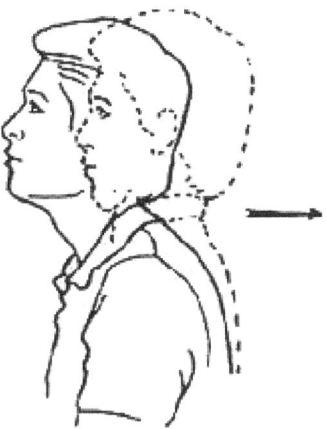

- **Chinning -** The starting position is the same as in previous two exercises place your head in its natural level and look straight ahead, then inhale and tuck in your chin. Afterword exhale and stick out your chin. You should repeat this movement 3-5 times, and remember to breathe. This exercise helps strengthening your neck muscles and keeping your head in a right position.

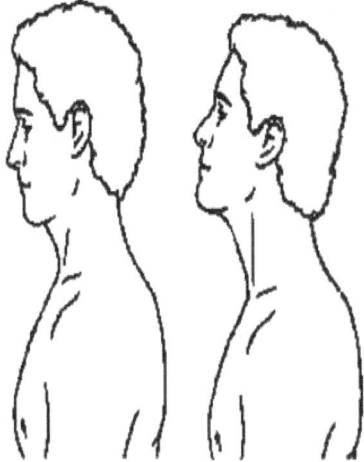

- **Shoulder shrug -** Keep your arms relaxed by your body. Lift your shoulders towards your ears. Squeeze your shoulder blades and rotate your shoulders to the back and then down to the starting position. Repeat this exercise 10 times. You should keep in mind that you should never rotate your shoulders forwards.

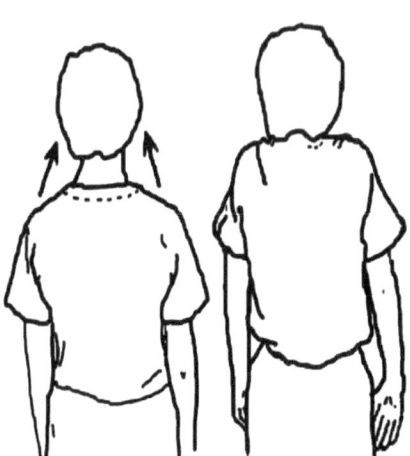

- **Shoulders retraction -** Touch your fingers to your ears and slightly raise your elbows. All the time remember not to push or pull on the neck. Squeeze your shoulder blades together. Stay in this position for 5 seconds and then release.

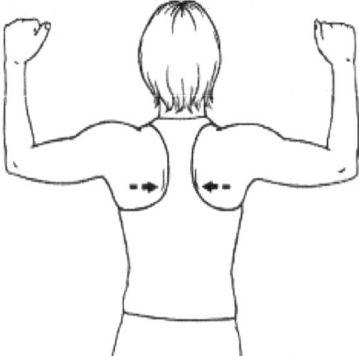

- **Upper back stretch.** Extend your arms in front of your body, clasp your hands together. Pull your shoulder blades apart gently, and then drop your chin to your chest. Hold this position for 10-30 seconds. Repeat this movement 10 times.

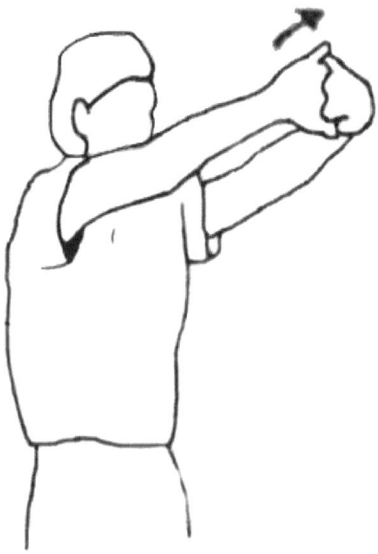

Neck muscles that run from the upper and middle neck down to the lower neck and shoulder blades are usually the initial cause of tension headaches, and stretching them will help you reduce the pain and keep your head pain free. If you feel that you would benefit more from customized exercises you should ask your doctor for tips or physical therapy.

Like with any other type of exercises you should remember to stay consistent and stick to your routine. These exercises will take 10-20 minutes of your daily free time, but in return you will live a life without constant headaches which tire and frustrate you.

Diet for preventing headaches

Research has shown that there are some proven ways in preventing the headaches by adjusting your diet plan. Vitamin b2 is one of the headache killers; it reduces the problem for up to 50%. This ingredient improves your brain metabolism and its muscles cells, which helps the brain in maintaining the much needed energy. Food rich in b2 is for example crimini mushrooms or asparagus, or to keep it simple a glass of low-fat milk. There are also diet supplements containing vitamin b2.

It is mentioned that women suffer from headaches more often than man. It is believed that the estrogen level can trigger this condition. In this case magnesium is helpful if you experience headaches on monthly basis. Try to add 450 mg of magnesium to your daily diet. Spinach is a rich source of this element, also Swiss chard. Besides this two there are some more foods containing magnesium, but in smaller amounts, such as sweet potatoes, bananas, sunflower seeds and sesame seeds.

You should add coenzyme Q10 which you can find in mackerel and tuna, broccoli and cauliflower. To get the best results be sure to get at least 100 mg of Q10 on the daily basis. This coenzyme is a rich source of energy production and therefore it is important for keeping your blood vessels healthy. Besides, it is a very powerful antioxidant. By eating food rich with this coenzyme you will protect your body from stress-induced free radicals.

While this as a basis for your new headache killer diet you should only add water-rich fruit like watermelon, strawberries, grapefruit or pineapple. Remember to stay hydrated, because it is very important to maintain the water balance in your organism. Also, you should remember to avoid smoking, exaggerating with alcohol and caffeine. There are some foods that are proven to affect the severity of headaches, so you should try to minimize the usage of this food in your everyday nutrition plan. Those are: dairy, chocolate, peanut butter, fruits such as avocado and banana, meat with nitrates, such as hot dogs and bacon, basically any over processed food.

Homeopathic treatment

In this part you will learn how to treat your headaches naturally, by home-made homeopathic remedies. There are some herbs and cures that were proven successful in addressing the problem of headaches and migraines. If you want to treat your condition avoiding chemical treatment then you should try out these natural cures that do not have side effects and can significantly improve your overall health status.

- **Lavender Oil.** Lavender oil is known for its great impact on health and different condition. The herb smells great and what is most important it is proven that lavender oil can reduce headaches. You can inhale it or apply it topically, that is on you to decide which way suits your needs best. If you choose to inhale the herb, pour 2-3 drops of the oil in the same amount of cups of boiling water. You should inhale the evaporating water, whilst covered by a towel, or something similar. Unlike other medical oils, you can apply it directly to your skin without diluting it. It is not recommended to use the herb orally.

- **Peppermint Oil.** Peppermint is a soothing home remedy that has been shown to benefit avoiding different types of headaches, especially tension headaches. This has a vaso-constricting and vaso-dilating properties, which helps in controlling a healthy blood flow through your organism. We have mentioned before that headaches can appear as a result of a poor blood flow. It is now clear how the peppermint oil has a great impact on this types of headaches. Also, because of the sharp smell, this oil opens up the sinuses. Corked sinuses are often a reason for headaches, so opening them up is a crucial step in treating this type of headaches.

- **Basil oil.** Basil is a great choice for tension headaches because it works as a muscle relaxant. Exercises that help you relax your tense muscles in combination with this oil are a great home remedy. You can use the oil to massage the stiff areas of your neck in order to relax.

- **Feverfew -** Feverfew is used to reduce the bodily temperature, but it is also good in helping to relieve headaches. There are studies that prove that feverfew is best to be taken on daily basis, especially in combination with white willow, which contains properties similar to aspirin, but without any harmful side effects.

- **Flaxseed** - Omega 3 fatty acids, stored in flaxseed, can reduce headaches provoked by different types of inflammation processes. You can use it in different forms, ranging from oil to whole seed.

- **Apple cider vinegar**. This ingredient has a long history as a successful natural remedy. It's been used to relieve everything from scurvy to hay fever. Some modern day studies have proven its effectiveness in treating certain illnesses, but most of its clout lies in the reports of people throughout the centuries who have benefited from it. This remedy will help improving your circulation and you will benefit a lot from it. Try to drink it with water every morning and you will notice the results in improving your overall health, but especially headaches.

Besides this most used remedies there are a lot of other cures that you can try out, for example cayenne pepper, fish oil, gingerroot etc. Basically anything that helps your blood flow and that helps you relax will be a useful way in treating your problem.

Remember living a healthy life and changing of your everyday habits is a successful key in getting rid of headaches, or any other problem of modern man living in a stressful society. Sleep enough, eat healthy, exercise and avoid chemical treatment, unless you really have to use it. With a more relaxed point of view, and caring for your body it is guaranteed you will achieve great results in maintaining a healthy and active life long into future.

Conclusion

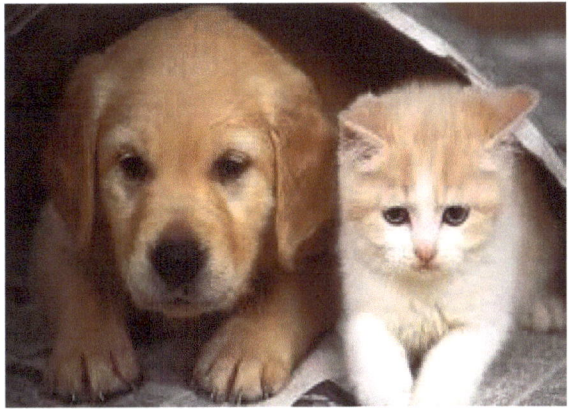

Before you go, I'd like to say thank you for purchasing my book.

I know you could have picked so many other books to read on pain management. But you took a chance on me.

So A Big thanks for downloading this book and reading it all the way to completion.

Now I would like to ask a _small_ favor.

Could you please take a minute or two to leave a review for this book on Amazon?

Click here

The feedback will help me continue to publish more kindle books that will help people to get better results in their lives.

And if you found it helpful in anyway then please let me know :-)

The Arthritis Pain Cure

How To Find Arthritis Pain Relief And Live A Happy Pain Free Life

By

Michele Gilbert

<u>Visit My Amazon Author Page</u>

Introduction

I want to thank and congratulate you for downloading the book, *"The Arthritis Pain Cure; How To Find Arthritis Pain Relief And Live A Happy Pain Free Life"*

This book contains proven steps and strategies on how to make your life with arthritis more comfortable and how to relieve the pain.

If you want to find out how to relieve the pain that arthritis brings, you have downloaded the right book. In this book you will learn about the comprehensive ways to cope with your condition. Addressing the problem from different angles is the best way to take your life back into your own hands and start enjoying it to the fullest. Take your time, get informed and start helping yourself!

Thanks again for downloading this book, I hope you enjoy it!

Chapter 1

What is Arthritis?

Arthritis is a condition provoked by the inflammation of joints and is very common among people aged fifty-five and older. It is a mundane health problem that affects one in every five American adults. The most common types of arthritis are osteoarthritis and rheumatoid arthritis. To better understand what happens with your body if you have the condition, I will first explain the structure of the joint. The joint is the crossing from one bone to another connected with ligaments which hold the bones in place. Because the bones are not directly leaning against each other there is a natural linker called cartilage that covers the bone surface. Cartilage is the essential joint component that allows the joints to work painlessly and smoothly. The joint is surrounded by synovial fluid which nourishes the joint and the cartilage. Depending on what type of arthritis you have, some of the parts of the joint will be affected and will prevent the joint from working properly. The causes of the disease vary; ranging from genetics, injuries and obesity to infections.

The signs and symptoms of arthritis also vary depending on which type of condition is responsible. Symptoms of *Osteoarthritis* develop slowly and gradually. When it comes to this type of the condition, the most affected areas of the body are the spine, hips, knees and hands. For every type of arthritis, the patient will find it hard to move and will feel pain in the joints. There may be swelling and the person will feel the joints are stiff, especially in the morning. *Rheumatoid* arthritis causes the same bodily sensations as the previous type, differing only in the fact that this type of arthritis spreads from smaller to bigger joints and results in it affecting the whole body, even the jaw, when not treated. Rheumatoid arthritis can cause the feeling of tiredness and fatigue and could also lead to weight loss. The dominant symptom of *Infectious* arthritis is fever, followed by pain and joint swelling. In most cases only one joint is affected.

Arthritis affects people in different ways, depending on the type and severity. Still, it doesn't matter how much you suffer, the condition limits you from doing your daily routine and you probably feel frustrated. If you want to get your life back in your hands, this book is made for you, to help you ease your pain and maintain the active daily routine you had before the arthritis came into your life!

Chapter 2

Chemical Therapy

Chemical therapy is the first choice that comes to mind when thinking about relieving pain. The choice of which drug suits you best for treating the condition, you should leave to your doctor. Still, there are some drugs that can help you relieve the pain. These drugs are known as analgesics and are actually the combination of drugs made to help you ease the ache. Some of these drugs can be bought without prescription and these can be simple pain killers as paracetamol. Also, you could use non-steroidal and anti-inflammatory drugs as aspirin and ibuprofen. Some forms of arthritis are treated with steroid therapy which can be administered in the form of tablets or injections. The others that can only be purchased with the prescription of your doctor belong to the category of narcotics. You should be careful with using these, because they can cause an addiction which can lead to the result that the drug becomes more and more ineffective on the user. On the market, you can also find biological response modifiers, which are created in laboratory and used in treating severe forms of arthritis. These medications have a lot of side-effects and are to be used only with the strict supervision of your doctor. What is commonly used for treating the disease are Gold salts which come in the form of Gold thioglucose known as *solganal* and gold thiomalate known as myochrysine administered in the form of an injection. Gold salts are also made in the form of an oral drug, auronafin, known as *ridaura*. These drugs can also cause unpleasant side-effects.

If you want to try out the chemical treatment, you should consult your doctor before doing it. Still, in some cases that are not extremely severe, maybe the best choice is to try out alternative ways of treating the condition. The drugs address the problem directly, but, because your body functions as a machine and each part of your immune system is interconnected, the best way to treat the problem is holistically, from different angles.

Chapter 3

Physical Therapy

The biggest problem that most of the patients with arthritis face is their immobility and the pain they are feeling which is stopping them in their active life, limiting their movement. This situation can be frustrating because it alters the way that individuals are used to carrying out their daily routine. Another crucial step in your process of relieving pain and treating the condition is physical therapy. The symptom of stiff joints is actually caused by avoiding physical activity because of the pain provoked by movement. So the benefits of physical therapy are clear; by favoring an active life you are actually helping yourself to eliminate the pain you feel and problems you are facing.

Being passive and inactive will not help you cope with your condition. Exercise is a crucial part of your process of getting better, but it has to be done consistently, every day and you have to do it right. Also, the physical activity will help you lose weight which is very important in treating arthritis, because every pound lost is four pound less pressure on your joints, especially the knees.

There are some crucial things you should keep in mind. Foremost, you should consult an experienced physical therapist who will make an individualized program that will be based on your condition. Your therapist should monitor your progress and give you guidelines to help you beat the arthritis. **Never give up!** Like with every other exercise it is likely that you will get tired, frustrated and that you will not see the results immediately. With a help of your therapist and positive thinking you can do a lot. Do not make up excuses.

Remember, you want to be mobile, active and feel better. Sometimes you will feel the pain that you cannot cope with, but still keep working out, focus on a different part of the body, or change the type of movement. Find what best suits you and keep up. If you are facing a problem of stiff joints, use a warm shower. Heat increases blood supply to the hurting area and relieves the pain. Warm shower will also help you feel relaxed. The aerobic exercises have shown great results and what is most important, you can do them on your own, they are not expensive and you can make them fun. Do whatever you want, from walking with your friends or dog to swimming, whatever suits you best. Just be careful with the amount of working out and do not exceed the limits of your ability. Set up your goals; find the reason to make yourself feel better. When you feel discouraged and when you have a bad day just repeat your goals. Do not be ashamed or afraid to ask for help and support. Your friends and family are there for you. You have to keep in mind that you are not alone in this; there are millions of people throughout the world that are feeling the way you do. You can also find out if there is a support group for your condition so you can share your experience with someone who is facing the same difficulties. It is always easier to feel the comfort of someone who understands you.

Chapter 4

Diet for Arthritis

The changing of your diet is not going to help you relieve the pain, but it will most certainly affect your overall health and lower the inflammation. You will not feel the results immediately, but with time, if you keep focusing attention on what you eat, your overall condition will improve. Remember, there is not an immediate solution to your problems and you should not look for it. You have to acquire the habits that will improve the quality of your life. Foods related to the Mediterranean diet slows down the inflammation process.

So there are some ingredients that you should use as often as possible.

- **Fish -** Fish contains omega-3 fatty acids that are good for reducing inflammation. Besides that, omega-3 will affect your overall health because it reduces blood fat and also helps keep away depression and dementia. The best choice in fishes for you include: herring, salmon, sardines, tuna and lake trout. If you just don't like the taste of fish, good substitutes are walnuts, flaxseed and soybean oil.
- **Olive oil -** Olive oil contains oleocanthal which reduces arthritis inflammation. Try and replace the fats you are using in your everyday nutrition with olive oil. The health benefits of olive oil are great. Besides stopping the inflammation, olive oil preserves your heart, prevents stroke, and more importantly for women, it lowers the risk of breast cancer.
- **Fruits and Vegetables -** Fruits and vegetables decrease the enzymes that cause inflammation because they contain antioxidants and phytochemicals. If you want to improve your diet in order to preserve your health and keep the symptoms under control you should eat more apples and citrus fruits and also red and yellow onions, potatoes and ginger.
- **Whole grains -** You should eat cereals and whole grain breads. Whole grains can also lower the risk of a stroke, risk of heart disease and helps you maintain a healthy weight. They will give you more energy, so you could do your physical therapy more effectively.

Chapter 5

Acupuncture

The point of acupuncture is to restore the balance of energy in the body. Acupuncture is the Chinese practice that can be traced back 2500 years. It is a procedure that is based on stimulating anatomical locations in the skin by inserting stainless needles. According to traditional Chinese medical theory Gi - vital energy flows through the body which is divided into meridians. Acupuncture is the process of stimulating these meridians through which the vital energy flows and the goal is to restore the balance of energy because the body is only healthy if everything is in harmony. Acupuncture is thought to decrease pain by increasing the endorphins which block the pain. Releasing of endorphins blocks the transmission of the pain from the nerves to the brain.

Acupuncture is the best way of treating chronic pain, and arthritis is exactly that. Even though the needles are inserted in your skin in acupuncture treatment, you will feel only a slight prick, much lighter than what is felt when you are receiving an injection.

After the treatment you will probably feel heaviness and mild soreness. If the treatment is done right, the process is completely safe because it is done with sterile disposable needles.
It is on you to find a competent practitioner and get well informed about the process and conditions of performing the treatment. The biggest advantage of this approach to treating your condition is that it is completely drug-free. With drugs, it is common that people develop tolerance to drugs after prolonged usage often resulting in a need for increase dosage and drug dependence. The other advantage is that the number of treatments is individualized as done by professionals in this field who will examine you and assess the state of your illness.

Chapter 6

Homeopathic Treatment

Homeopathic approach is based on looking at a person as a whole. Foremost the treatment starts with detecting the problem in few steps: What is it? Where is it? How long has it there? The most important step is detecting the evolution of the problem, which basically entails finding out where it started and what happened further along; are there any patterns of progressing? For successful treatment, your therapist should look for modalities which means that s/he has to be able to notice the causes that triggers you to feel better or worse. Also, a thorough anamnesis could be the clue to address your problems. A good homeopathic treatment should also involve the investigation of your mental status, to see how you cope with difficulties that the disease may have caused.

There are some herbs that have proven to help with treating arthritis. So I will make a list for you.

- **Aloe Vera** - This herb is one of the most extensively used herbs in alternative medicine. Due to its well known health benefits in managing different types of conditions, it is also used in relieving arthritis pain. The Aloe Vera gel can be applied on the skin at aching joints. If used orally it can have some side-effects, but if used topically, it is completely safe.
- **Boswellia** - This herb is known for its anti-inflammatory effect. This herb is available in the form of a tablet and as a topical cream. It is safer to try out the cream because medical research has not fully ascertained how it affects humans when ingested.
- **Cat's claw** - This herb may help reduce swelling at the joints. It works by improving the immune system. With this herb, you have to be careful with dosage because it could overstimulate the immune system potentially leading to the worsening of arthritis symptoms.
- **Eucalyptus** - Eucalyptus is widely available in western markets. You can find and purchase it easily. The leaves contain tannins which are proven to be helpful in treating swelling and hence the reduction of pain. It is best used in topical cream form.
- **Ginger -** Ginger is known for its anti inflammatory properties. The best way to use this plant that you probably have at your home is to cook a fresh tea out of it and drink it every morning. This herb will do your overall health good.
- **Green tea -** Green tea is used to reduce inflammation of the body, so it is clear how it can help you with your problem. Besides that, it has a lot of other health benefits. It reduces blood cholesterol and it lowers the potential risk of a heart disease which is known to affect arthritis patients.

This list was created to offer you help with coping with arthritis. Still, you have to be aware that you should consult a specialist before using any of these products because every organism is unique and something that works on others may not work on you.

Chapter 7

Topical Pain Medication

When the feeling of pain associated with arthritis continues even after you have taken your drugs, then it is perhaps best to use some cream, gel or patch that will help you ease the ache. Topical medications are absorbed through your skin and are the best solution for avoiding extra medication. Because the ingredients are absorbed through the skin they are most effective on the joints where the skin is thin and near to the bones as in case of knees and fingers.

The most helpful ingredients used in these kinds of products are **capsaicin, salycilates** and **counterirritants.** Capsaicin causes burning sensations and works on the basis of stopping the nerve cells from sending the pain message to the nervous system. Salycilates contain the ingredients that are used for aspirin. Counterirritants cause the sensation of heat or coldness that can stop your ability to feel the pain. Most common substances are menthol and camphor.

A lot of people are satisfied with the effects of these products and most importantly they are safe for use if used properly. You should wash your hands thoroughly after applying the creams and contact with the eyes because of the burning sensation they produce. If your skin is sensitive, you may use latex gloves when applying the cream or gel.

Chapter 8

Electrical Stimulation

This is one of the interventions that could be used in treating arthritis. There are different types of electrical stimulation ranging from muscle tissue stimulation to strengthening of muscle tissue that supports the affected joint. This way of treating the pains caused by the condition is used only if other ways prove to be inefficient.

The technique used is called transcutaneous electrical nerve stimulation (TENS). In this method of treatment, a small device that sends mild electric pulses through electrodes placed around the aching area in order to stimulate the nerves is used. This type of treatment like some others described in this book helps in blocking the pain message.

This procedure is not painful but it may cause a tingling sensation.

Chapter 9

Chiropractic Treatment

Most patients that have tried chiropractic practices in treating arthritis pain were very satisfied. Some professionals think that the chiropractic treatment should be an additional treatment for arthritis, especially in the case of the most common form of the condition, osteoarthritis.

Chiropractic is an approach that focuses on disorder of the musculoskeletal system and the nervous system which causes a lot of health related issues. The biggest advantage of this approach is that it is completely drug-free and it is based on hands-on approach to health care. For this to be done right, you should, as in every case consult a professional that will examine you and pay attention to your disease history. The measures to be taken are to be individualized so they can suit every patient.

It is shown that a lot of patients feel relief only after three chiropractic treatments. It is better to take a long-term approach to your healing, because every case is different and your goal here is to get rid of the pain caused by arthritis for as long as possible. The number of treatments depends on your condition and on what your goals for accessing this treatment are.

In chiropractic, different approaches are used. Gentle manipulation techniques are used to help reduce the stiffness you feel. In this mode of treatment, different types of massages and exercises are used. Massage increases blood flow and brings warmth to the sore joint. Also, if needed, you can ask for low level laser treatment, inferential and ultrasound practices, but the professional will know what suits you best.

Chapter 10

Nutritional Supplements

The most commonly used and effective supplements that you could add to your daily routine are glucosamine and chondroitin. These supplements are the components of a normal cartilage. The effect provoked by using these supplements is the stimulation of the body to produce more cartilage. The products you can find in pharmacies are the ones that are tested and safe. Still, if you are using any type of medicine for your condition, you should consult your doctor because these supplements could limit the effect of other drugs if used in the wrong way.

Conclusion

In treating arthritis you should understand that pain is not completely a bodily sensation. The pain is tightly connected to your state of mind and can be produced in the mental and emotional realm. So to threat the pain you should not focus all attention only to your body, you should try and train your mind. Also, you should keep in mind that pain is only the sign; it is basically an alarm that your body has set to warn you about the condition. So in treating the pain, the most effective way is to find the root of the problem and treat them holistically so you can eliminate your aches and keep the symptoms under control. Still, because arthritis pain is a chronic pain and controlling this type of pain is essential so you can keep up with your everyday routine undisturbed, pain treatments may be necessary while holistic treatment is ongoing.

Your attitude towards pain is crucial to how you react and cope with it. You should admit that you have pain and take actions to relieve it. **You should take control** and you should be aware that the mind is playing an important role in how you perceive this pain and how in turn you cope with it. There are some tips that could help you control the aches emotionally.

You should keep a positive attitude. Do not build your life around your pain and do not let it control you. This condition can limit you, but it should never control your life. If you realize that you are the master of your life, then you will be stronger than the pain you feel.
You should constantly remind yourself about things that you can do. Do them and enjoy doing it, not torturing yourself with thoughts about the things you are not able to do. Do not think about your pain, keep yourself distracted by doing things you like, spending time with people you love and enjoying your life to the fullest.

You should remember that you are not alone in this. If you tend to forget this and feel lonely, seek a support group that will help you communicate what you feel because communication is important when dealing with any form of discomfort. Ask for help when you need it. Learn how to overcome your problem with sharing your experience with other people.

Relax more and avoid stress. Relax and consider learning ways to calm and control your body. Don't be over anxious. With a little bit of practice and getting to know your body, you will learn how to relax and beat the aches you are feeling.

Live a healthy life. Take your medication, change your diet, exercise and don't let the pain control you!

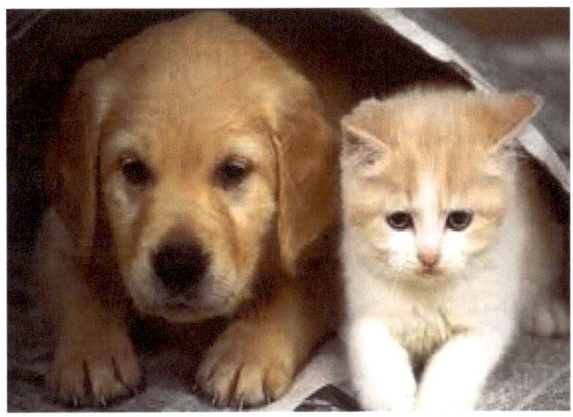

Thank you again for downloading this book!

.

Before you go, I'd like to say thank you for purchasing my book.

I know you could have picked so many other books to read about Pain Relief. But you took a chance on me.

So A Big thanks for downloading this book and reading it all the way to completion.

Now I would like to ask a _small_ favor.

Could you please take a minute or two to leave a review for this book on Amazon?

Click here

Preview of My New Book

Adrenal Fatigue: What Is Adrenal Fatigue Syndrome And How To Reset Your Diet And Your Life

CHAPTER 1
So What Is Adrenal Fatigue

Get used to the idea right away that even if your symptoms fit like a glove, a good many people, including doctors, may tell you there is no such thing as Adrenal Fatigue. There are illnesses which share the symptoms, and you should rule those out first. The chances are, though, that you have picked this book because you've had all the tests, you've been cleared as healthy—and yet you still feel as though healthy and active is a dim and distant memory. The best thing to do next is learn as much as you can about Adrenal Fatigue. You picked the right book!

The following sections are designed to tell you the symptoms and causes of the syndrome, those likeliest to have it, the lifestyle triggers for it (and managing or changing them), the traditional and homeopathic approaches, adjusting your diet, and ways of tackling the problem generally. One thing is for sure, nothing in this book can do other than help. That's important, because some of the supplements and vitamins marketed to treat Adrenal Fatigue aren't necessarily safe, and can have the opposite effect, causing your adrenal glands more distress. Treatments can also be expensive, because medical insurance won't usually cover them.

Before you could skip straight to the next section, with the signs and symptoms, you should learn what adrenal fatigue is.

The adrenal glands are walnut-sized, situated above each kidney, and react swiftly to help you cope with difficult situations. They were originally designed to flood our systems with the boost we needed in emergencies, but the problem with modern life is that the brain is constantly reacting to what it sees as emergency situations. Stress, handled properly, is actually essential to our survival but when the button is pressed too often, triggering a body response time and again, the glands go into overdrive, or they malfunction.

There are two of them and when they are working normally they provide, in lay terms, adrenaline (the fight-or-flight hormone), noradrenaline (which reacts to fear and affects blood pressure), cortisol (which plays a role in blood sugar management and your immune system) dopamine (affecting your nervous central system) and steroids. They are essential to our wellbeing and balance. Healthy adrenal gland secretions have us feeling at our strongest and most alert at the start of the day, tapering off naturally towards the end of the day, so that we fall asleep easily, wake feeling rested, and have energy to call on.

Constant or intense stress, or respiratory infections, even a serious attack of 'flu, can affect their performance and leave you feeling tired, unwell, depressed and generally off-color. When this gray feeling can't be shaken off and becomes chronic, yet medical tests can't pick up any physical cause, you have a classic Adrenal Fatigue profile. It probably isn't any consolation, but you share that profile with millions of others.

CHAPTER 2
What Are The Signs and Symptoms of Adrenal Fatigue

It has been referred to as the 21st century stress disorder, and is often dismissed by the medical profession. In fairness to them, changes to the adrenal glands can be too slight to be picked up in medical tests, despite the impact even slight changes have to the body. To anyone suffering it, the changes may be medically slight, but they have a devastating effect on lifestyle, especially as it often affects people who eat healthily, exercise, and keep themselves in shape, yet are increasingly fatigued.

If you have several of the following symptoms, there are tests that will pick up the more alarming alternatives, listed at the end of this section. Have them done.

Stop Back Pain NOW!

Back Pain Remedies And Treatments To Live A Pain Free Life

By

Michele Gilbert

Dedicated to those who choose to stretch beyond their own limits and to seek a more abundant and fulfilling life

Your thoughts are creative.

Michele Gilbert

My Free Gift To You!

As a way of saying thank you for downloading my book, I am willing to give you access to a selected group of readers who (every week or so) receive inspiring, life-changing kindle books at deep discounts, and sometimes even absolutely free.

Wouldn't it be great to get amazing Kindle offers delivered directly to your inbox?

Wouldn't it be great to be the first to know when I'm releasing new fresh and above all sharply discounted content?

But why would I do something like this?

Why would I offer my books at such a low price and even give them away for free when they took me countless hours to produce?

Simple…. Because I Want To Spread The Word.!

For a few short days Amazon allows Kindle authors to promote their newly released books by offering them deeply discounted (up to 70% price discounts and even for free. This allows us to spread the word extremely quickly allowing users to download thousands and thousands of copies in a very short period of time.

Once the timeframe has passed, these books will revert back to their normal selling price. That's why you will benefit from being the first to know when they can be downloaded for free!

So are you ready to claim your weekly Kindle books?

You are just one click away! Follow the link below and sign up to start receiving awesome content

Thank you and Enjoy!

Introduction

I want to thank you and congratulate you for downloading the book, *"Stop Back Pain Now; Back Pain Remedies and Treatments so you can live a pain free life!"*

This book contains proven steps and strategies on how to make your life with back pain more comfortable, but also how to prevent the condition from developing.

In this book we are offering detailed explanation on different causes and types of back pain. Also, in order to keep your life drug-free we have represented different alternative treatments that you could consider. For mild forms of back pain there are some DIY techniques that will help you in keeping your life pain-free, but also preventing back pain conditions to develop.

Thanks again for downloading this book, I hope you enjoy it!

What is back pain?

The most important step in treating any health-related problem you are experiencing is to get to know the problem. Back pain is a very common complaint. It is estimated that 80% of Americans will experience lower back pain sometimes in their lives. In United Kingdom back pain is the most common reason for absence from the workplace. This problem is mostly very painful, but it is not a serious health problem. Back pain can range from dull, constant ache, to a sudden, sharp pain that makes you paralyzed and unable to move. Still, you do not need to live in pain, learn how to get rid of it and continue with your day-to-day activities pain free and satisfied.

Pain in the back may be linked to the bony lumbar spine, discs between the vertebrae, ligaments around the spine and discs, spinal cord and nerves, lower back muscles, abdomen, internal organs, but also the skin around the lumbar area.

The risk factor that could effect on the development of back pain is:

- Stressful job
- Pregnant women are more likely to develop back pain
- If you spend your day mostly in sedentary position you are more likely to develop back pain condition
- Older adults are more susceptible than children or young people
- Anxiety
- Depression
- Back pain is most common among women
- If you are obese, the pressure on the bones is stronger so you are likely to have back pain problems
- Smoking stops the flow of nutrients to the disks in your back, that`s why you could develop back pain condition.
- Intensive physical exercise, especially if not done right, can be a cause for this problem
- Poor physical fitness is also a common cause of this condition.
- Intensive physical work. If you have to lift and pull things as part of your job.
- Some causes of back pain, for example ankylosing spondylitis, a form of arthritis can be genetically related.

Causes of back pain

In most cases back pain is caused by some physical injury or, on the other hand, as a result of specific condition of your bones or muscles. The human back is composed of a complex structure of bones, ligaments, muscles and nerves that are interconnected, if one part does not function properly you will experience pain that will block your motion range and cause troubles in doing things that you are used to. Pain that is caused from the muscle spasm can be severe and intensive, but pain provoked by the number of different syndromes can become chronic and it has to be treated properly.

Back pain is extremely mundane but the severity and symptoms can vary a lot. A simple pain caused by muscle strain can cause an excruciating pain that can lead you to the emergency room. Degenerating disc, or another condition, can cause constant and mild pain, that people often ignore, seeing it only as something that will stop and ignoring the symptoms, but this problem needs to be professionally addressed so the development of chronic health problem is avoided.

As with any other health related problem, on-time and precise defining the symptom is the crucial step in treating the problem and choosing a right treatment for pain relief.

Exercise program for back pain relief

In the previous text you have find out that back pain comes with age. Ensuring a pain-free life is same as any other investment in the future. If you develop a back pain problem you won`t be able to enjoy in anything you have accomplished. That is why we are offering an easy exercise plan that will prevent the condition to appear, but also, if the pain started help you relief it. As with any other exercise plan you have to be consistent in what you are doing so you can see the results. Throw away the excuses and start working on your health in order to live a pain free life.

With this program you do not need any additional exercise equipment and also access to gym, you can do the exercises whilst watching television, or taking a break from your other daily activities. It is crucial that you commit to the program, but consider it as something fun.

The following are stretches that aid in pain relief and may help, also, in stopping the advancement of arthritis. These exercises should be done pain-free, do not force your body on something you are not able to do. If you start experiencing pain while doing the program stop and take a break.

- **Piriformis Muscle Stretching Exercise**

The *piriformis* muscle runs from the thigh bone to the base of the spine. To stretch these muscles you have to lie on your back and cross the painful leg over the other. Bent your knees and place the hands under the lower leg and slowly pull the bottom leg towards the chest. You should stay in this position for about 30 seconds, while keeping the both legs closely until the stretching is felt. Remember do not jerk the legs or do any forced movement, does it gently. If you are experiencing pain you have probably done something wrong. Repeat this movement couple of times. Do the exercise 1-2 times a day.

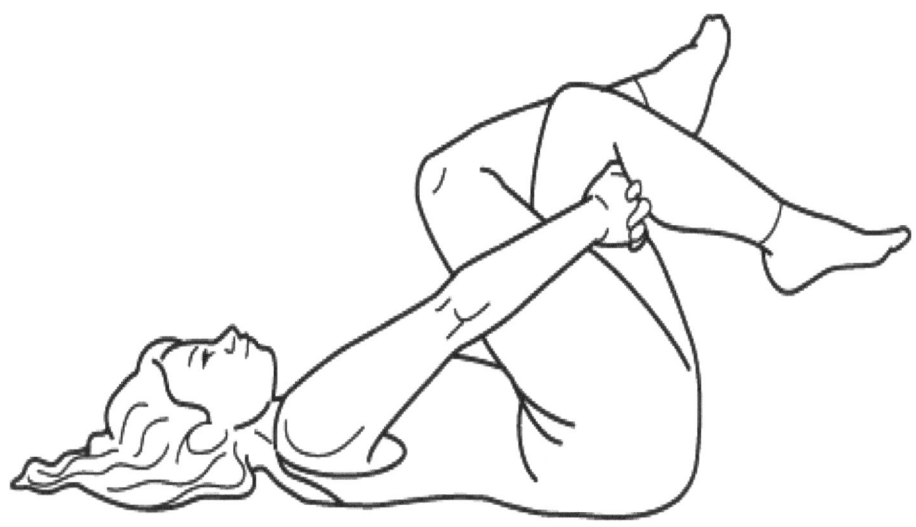

- **Psoas Major Muscle Stretching Exercise**

The *psoas major* muscle is attached to the front portion of lower back spine and can limit your movement ability when tight and sore. If you have difficulty of standing a long period of time or kneeling, than you probably have a problem with this muscle. This muscle can be stretched when you are kneeling on one knee. When you are in this position, rotate the free leg outward and keep tight the gluteal muscles on the side you are stretching. When you have done this, lean forward, but use the hips, not the lower back. You should feel a stretch in the front side of the hip that you are kneeling on. As in the previous exercise hold in this position 30 seconds, repeat as you feel comfortable and perform this movement 1-2 times a day.

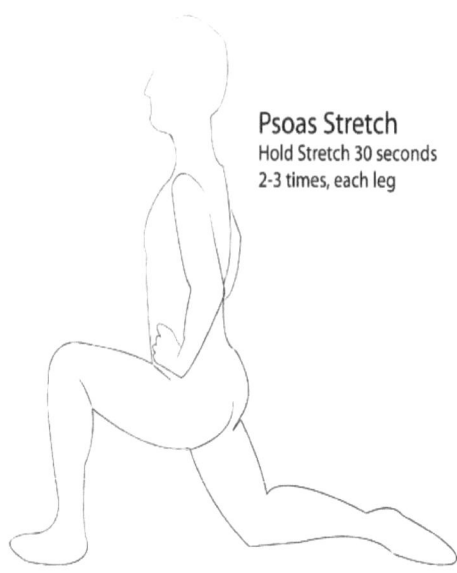

Psoas Stretch
Hold Stretch 30 seconds
2-3 times, each leg

- **Hamstring Muscle Stretching Exercise**

The *hamstring muscle* runs from the pelvic bone to the back of the knee. These muscles control the movement of bending the knee and flexing the gluteal muscles in order to extend the hip. These muscles are really important to stretch because they make possible the sitting in a straight up position. People who do not sit properly, straight up, are at risk of developing degenerative disk condition that is why you should work on stretching these muscle groups, to prevent the condition, but also to ease the pain if you have developed a disease. To perform this exercise you should lay on your back, grasp the leg behind the knee with the hip flexed to 90 degrees and the knee slightly bent. The most important movement is to straighten the knee whilst keeping the toes pointed towards you. You should feel the stretching in the back part of your leg.

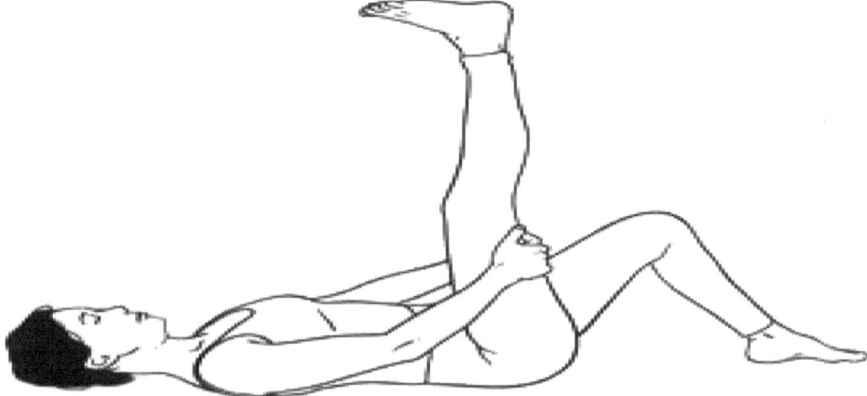

The exercises presented here were the stretching postures and movements that cannot do you any harm if you are doing them right. As we have recommended, do not cross the boundary of pain. The pain is an alarm that your body is sending you, which notices you that you are doing something that is not good for it. If you accept this exercise routine you will address the most important muscles that are the cause of lower back pain, but you will also manage to keep yourself fit and stretched.

Acupuncture

With acupuncture you will secure yourself of the back pain caused by some chronic conditions. Acupuncture is the way of restoring the flow of energy in the body. By inserting stainless needles the anatomical locations are stimulated and pain is relieved. A lot of physicians do recommend acupuncture therapy with chronic back pain when the conventional way of treatment is not working. If you want to avoid chemical treating of pain, you should try out this alternative method. Talk to your doctor about this solution and find a help from a certified professional.

The inserting of needles stimulates the central nervous system which is responsible for processing the information about the pain. Also, this stimulation can provoke releasing the chemicals into the muscles and spinal cord which alter the sense of pain or provoke the pain-free state.

Some theories argue that acupuncture functions by:

- Speeding the flow of electromagnetic signals, which can stimulate the production and circulation of endorphins that are responsible for killing the pain.
- Triggering the release of natural opioids, that is responsible for lessening the pain and promoting sleep.
- Increasing the release of neurotransmitters and neurohormones that are affecting the nervous system and ease the pain.

If you decide to try this method you should do it with a trained professional to avoid the side-effects. But remember, acupuncture, because it is a natural way of treating the health related problems, has less side-effect then drugs.

Homeopathic treatment of back pain

In this book we are trying to offer you comprehensive ways in treating the back pain condition and relieving the symptoms you are feeling, but avoiding the chemical treatment, which can bring you current relief, with lots of side effects. Homeopathic treatment is based on addressing the symptoms naturally, with the help of the herbs.

Any condition can be treated homeopathically and so is with the back pain. We are going to present you a list of most common back pain treatments, but if you want to find something that will suit your needs you should contact a professional whom will prescribe the treatment based on your symptoms and needs.

- *Aesculus* - If you feel a pain in the lowest back area, and mostly when you are standing up, whilst the sitting position is pain-free this is the remedy for your condition. This remedy is especially powerful if the lower back pain is accompanied with venous congestion and hemorrhoids.
- *Arnica montana* - This cure will help you in relieving back pain cause by overexertion or mild trauma.
- *Bryonia* - This remedy is for the sharp back pain caused even by a slightest motion. This pain is caused even when coughing and it is mostly caused as the effect of injury.
- *Calcarea carbonica* - This remedy is most useful for a back pain caused by obesity. Chronic back pain can lead to inflammation and soreness that are followed by the chilly feeling. If you are experiencing this type of pain you should try with this natural remedy.
- *Calcarea phosphorica* - Stiffness and pain of the spinal muscles, especially in the upper back and neck can be reduced by using this remedy. Aching in the bones can be treated with this cure.
- *Natrum nuriaticum* - If you feel soreness when lying on something hard, this type of back pain is caused by emotional stress and anger, and *natrum nuricaticum* is a most effective cure in treating it.
- *Nux vomica* - If you have muscle cramps that are relieved by applying something warm on the painful spot, also if the pain is getting worse by night and if you are experiencing constipation, try this remedy out.

- *Rhus toxicodendron* - This cure is prescribed if you feel a neck or back pain when moving. The pain is worse when the initial movement is made, but it gradually gets better through continued movement. Person finds it hard to stand or lie still. This remedy in combination with hot showers and massage gives proven results.

- *Sulphur* - If you experience pain in slouching posture you should try this cure out. The pain gets worse when standing up for a long period of time. Warmth worsens the feeling of soreness.

There are a lot of other homeopathic cures on the market. If you decide to treat your condition naturally and without side effect that are often with chemical treatment, you should contact a professional, or try some of these remedies out. Because they do not have side effect you can try them out on your own and see what works best for you.

Massage therapy

If muscle spasm is the cause of your back problems than massage is the best way of relieving it. The spasm should relax as part of the response to the pressure applied on the sore and spastic muscle. If there is no physical response noticeable, the cause of the pain is inflammation and that problem should not be addressed through massage therapy. In order for therapy to be effective the treatment should last at least 6 weeks and include four massage treatments. If there is no improvement after two massages this way of treating the condition probably won't work at all. If you have severe back pain you should first contact your doctor, before deciding to try massaging therapy out.

Massage therapy is most effective when combined with other medical treatments, as chiropractic or physical therapy. Many massage therapists are actually a part of an interdisciplinary group of professionals that will work on your problem. The pain cause by muscle spasm is a result of ischemic muscle treatment, which means that muscle is lacking a proper blood flow. Because the muscle is deprived of proper blood flow the oxygen flow is also interrupted which causes the spasm, which then causes the pain. Massage actually helps bringing the needed blood and oxygen to the sore muscles that are afterwards relaxed and pain-free.

This therapy will feel painful at first but the situation will improve. What you should keep in mind is that communication with therapist is of the major importance. You should inform the person performing the massage if the pressure is too mild or too hard. Good therapist will respond accordingly in order to help you relieve the pain you are feeling. Following the massage therapy process any pain should fade after 24 to 36 hours. The tensed muscles should be completely relaxed in the course of 4-14 days.

If you are sure that the pain is cause by muscle spasm you could try the self massage treatment. It is the simplest and cheapest way of addressing the back pain problem. If you do not feel a severe pain a few moments of gentle rubbing the sore area could help you a lot. The pain triggering point should be rubbed with your fingertips, thumbs, fist or elbow depending how you can reach the area easily. If the painful spot is hard to reach you can use some household tools that will help you reach it, for example tennis ball. You should just press the painful knot and hold the position for 10-100 seconds, the pressure should be gentle. You can also try with kneading strokes, that can be circular or back and forth. The crucial thing about the massage, which is actually a conversation with your nervous system is how hard to press. The rule is hard enough to be satisfying, but mild enough not to feel any pain. Pressure that you are applying should be clear and directed exactly to the sore spot and you should feel relieved. For the basic self-massage, trust your instincts, rub where it hurts. In order to notice the results, rub the sore sport every day for at least 30 minutes without stopping. If you have released the trigger point you will feel the reduction in symptoms over the next several hours. If you start feeling more pain stop the treatment. If you do not feel any relief, try different techniques of applying pressure and find out what works for you.

This way of treating back pain is also drug free and without any side-effects when done right. Remember, if you have a mild back pain you can experiment in order to relieve yourself of the pain you are feeling. If the symptoms are severe you should reach out for professional help. For mild pain, the best combination is exercise, self-massage and homeopathy, which you can do on your own. If the pain is severe you can use these techniques also, but you should be monitored by professionals.

Chiropractic treatment

Chiropractic treatment involves hands-on spinal manipulation, based on the theory that proper musculoskeletal structure will enable the well-being of the whole organism. Manipulation is used in order to restore the pain-free mobility to the joints, especially after the traumatic events as different types of injuries. This way of treatment is used for a relieving the pain.

First step when visiting a chiropractic professional is to make an accurate medical history and research what causes the back pain. The treatment will be adjusted to the general condition of your body and the frequency of treatments will be determined individually. Many chiropractors will involve a nutrition plan for the condition and work with the help of different techniques as for example physical rehabilitation plan. The goals of chiropractic treatment are restoration the bodily functions that were interrupted due to the pain, but also preventing further injuries that can cause it. Spinal manipulation, which is the basic of chiropractic technique, is a safe and effective way in treating acute back pain, especially caused by physical injuries. Acute back pain is different than chronic back pain, it lasts shorter and the symptoms fade away on their own, but to prevent the possible complications and consequences, it is not bad to consider the option of consulting the chiropractic professional. This technique is proven to be helpful in treating neck pain and headaches.

Although rare there have been the cases where some conditions causing back pain, as herniated or slipped disc, worsened after this type of treatment. That is why the most important step regarding chiropractic care should be taking the thorough condition history. Besides the benefits and dangers with this treatment method that we have informed you about, there are some extra benefits that you should consider. Chiropractic adjustment may affect the chemistry of biological processes on a cellular level, which will improve your overall health.

Back pain relief diet

The most common cause of back pain is some sort of inflammation. If you want to relieve the pain caused by inflammation process you should consider adjusting your diet to the developed condition. There is some food that is good in stopping the inflammation process and some that will worsen your condition. We will now present the basics of an anti-inflammation diet plan that could help you in beating the condition you have.

The best way to avoid or ease the inflammation is the vegetables base diet. Besides veggies you should also include flax and chia seeds in your everyday nutrition plan. The meat is best to be replaced with omega-3 rich fish, like salmon, herrings or tuna. Some of the ingredients that are most commonly eaten in this type of diet are carrots, sweet potatoes, grapes, cherries, red wine and watermelon. Spices that you should use are basil, cinnamon, ginger, garlic, rosemary and oregano. To avoid the inflammation developing further, you should drink natural herb teas; green tea is best known for anti-inflammatory effect.

Remember to avoid: processed foods, fast foods and saturated fats. Do not eat white bread, past, white rice, sugary drinks, snacks, fried foods etc. Caffeine and alcohol won`t do you any good either.

In order to keep your bones healthy, and also pain free, do eat food rich in calcium or add some calcium supplements in your everyday diet.

Remember your active life? Remember how much you love to take walks, swim, run and hike? Remember the days when you did not feel the pain in motion?

You do not deserve to feel pain, nobody does. If you want to live a healthy, pain-free life, and not be constrained with a sore body than work on it. This book will help you ease the pain you are feeling, but also prevent the condition from developing. Back pain and muscle and bones problems come with ageing, they are not something uncommon, and it is a natural process of your life. But, you can do a lot of things to prevent the pain to develop and become chronic. You should stay active and stretch your muscles every day. Also, diet is a crucial point in preventing different types of condition. Overall healthy way of life will ensure you the quality time in the future. Invest in your body and health. Stay active and pain free. If you have developed the back pain problems due to different factors, then try the tips we have represented you. If you want to treat yourselves on your own, you can try out the homeopathic cures, exercises and self-massage. But, if the condition is chronic and causing severe pain then consult your doctor. Try to avoid the medication and find an alternative way in treating the condition. The key step is communication. Track your symptoms and what feels most comfortable for you. In consulting a professional with whom you will have a good communication is the key of solving your problem.

Stay positive, maintain your health and enjoy your active life now and in the future!

Conclusion

Thank you again for downloading this book!

I hope this book was able to help you to relieve the back pain you are feeling and also prevent you from developing the condition.

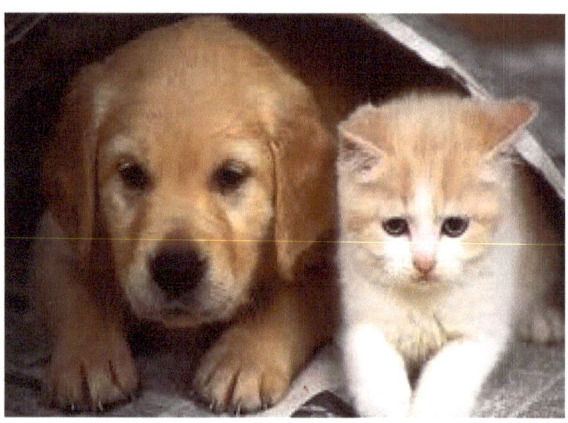

The next step is to take action!

I know you could have picked so many other books to read on Stopping Back Pain. But you took a chance on me.

So A Big thanks for downloading this book and reading it all the way to completion.

Now I would like to ask a *small* favor.

Could you please take a minute or two to leave a review for this book on Amazon?

Click here

The feedback will help me continue to publish more kindle books that will help people to get better results in their lives.

And if you found it helpful in anyway then please let me know :-)

Thank you and good luck!

Preview of My New Book

Body Language 101

What A Person's Body Language Is Really Telling You... And How You Can Use It To Your Advantage

Talk to the Hand

I don't know about you, but when I watch shows like *Lie to Me* or *Sherlock*, so often, I really, really wish that I could be that good. Heck, after I watched *The Mentalist* for the first time, I was studying everyone. I stared at footprints trying to see if I could tell whether the person walking was right handed or left handed. Not only is this super impractical for me as an actual skill, but it's super addicting. The thing is, it's all about studying people and watching them, but there's a science to it. I may not be out there catching criminals red handed for having a nervous tell, but it has helped me read situations and understand things that I previously missed.

So sure, you might not catch your arch-nemesis, but you might be able to understand things a little better with a little study of body language. And that's why I'm here. Body language is not just for detectives out there looking to catch murderers and thieves. Body language is the key to understanding the unspoken words that our body is communicating so heavily without our knowledge. Not only will this help you understand and relate to people better, but it'll make it so that you are aware of your own presence to others.

Nonverbal communication makes up the majority of our communication and most of us are clueless to the actual comprehension and understanding of it. That means that those who do not invest time in learning what to say in our nonverbal appearance are missing so much. But the truth is, we don't miss all of it. We have come to silently absorb and understand nonverbal communication, regardless of whether we know it or not. It's the art of learning to understand something we already know and to heighten our understanding and acceptance of what's being communicated to us. It's tricky, I know, but it's not impossible to understand.

What I'm going to tell you in this book is going to make sense to you and a lot of it is going to feel familiar, like you already knew that. Well, the reason for that is that you you've been picking up these silent transmissions for years, you just haven't acknowledged them or put a name to some of the habits you've already taught yourself.

So stick around and start to see if you can't agree or relate to some of the information you're going to receive. But more importantly, I want to address your homework before we start getting into the gritty, deep stuff. For instance, I want you to start watching people around you.

Observation is the birth of understanding and without a true sense of observance or a keen eye for noticing the little things, you're not going to pick up on some of these traits. When someone is talking to you, you're going to need to start watching them. Notice how they're standing, note the posture, have you looked at their eyes, what about the overall harmony of their face, and what are they doing with their hands? All of these things need to be running through your mind to really catch what is being conveyed to you. But not just watching their body, note the tones they're using, and the words that they're selecting. These are all going to tell you what sort of body language comes with certain attitudes and emotions. It all ties together and it is all relevant when it comes to understanding body language. So start opening your eyes and let's have a look at what they're trying to say to you.

Are you ready?

Weapons of Mass Induction

Though Sherlock Holmes often touts his use of deductive reasoning, it is actually the opposite that we're going to focus on with you, because right now, you're a student. For those of you that do not know, inductive reasoning starts with observations that slowly build a pattern that you will then form into a hypothesis until it is proven right or wrong. If you're right, then you have a theory.

For example, Kayla touches her hair a lot when she talks to Hot Mike, but not when she's talking to anyone else. So, every time I see Kayla talking to Hot Mike and she's touching her hair, that might be a cue that she likes Hot Mike. So, until I'm proven wrong, I'm certain that I have a theory that when a woman likes a man, she'll touch her hair unconsciously.

Viola, you have just jumped from observation to theory until proven wrong. Of course, when you're Sherlock Holmes level, you'll be using the art of deductive reasoning which starts at a theory and then tested with a hypothesis and observations until you have a conclusion. I think it's time for another example to prove this one to you.

Click Here To Read The Rest of

Body Language 101

What A Person's Body Language Is Really Telling You... And How You Can Use It To Your Advantage

P.S. You'll find many more books like this and others under my name Michele Gilbert.

Don't miss them… here is a short list.

Wicca: The Ultimate Beginners Guide For Witches and Warlocks: Learn Wicca Magic

The Introvert's Advantage: The Introverts Guide To Succeeding In An Extrovert World

Stop Playing Mind Games: How To Free Yourself Of Controlling And Manipulating Relationships

Instant Charisma: A Quick And Easy Guide To Talk, Impress, And Make Anyone Like You

Chakras: Understanding The 7 Main Chakras For Beginners: The Ultimate Guide To Chakra Mindfulness, Balance and Healing

Practicing Mindfulness: Living in the moment through Meditation: Everyday Habits and Rituals to help you achieve inner peace

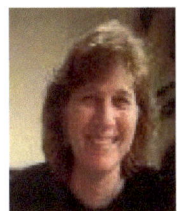

Michele Gilbert was born and raised in Brooklyn, New York. Drawn to literature and writing at a young age, she enrolled at Brooklyn College and majored in English. After graduation Michele did not begin writing immediately, instead she embarked on a career in the finance industry and spent the next thirty years on Wall Street.

Serendipity struck when she least expected it. After ending a long-term relationship, Michele found herself lost and unsure what the future held. She began to read books on grief and loss, looking for answers. Those led her to delve deeper into the Law of Attraction and its power. What resulted was remarkable. Not only had she begun to heal, she had also rekindled her former love of writing and discovered her life's purpose.

The years have taken her through many twists and turns, but she learned valuable lessons along the way. Today she publishes books-mostly self-help and metaphysical in nature-and feels compelled to share her knowledge with those facing similar experiences. Her greatest hope is to inspire others and show them ways to overcome adversity and gracefully accept life's inevitable low points.

Going forward, she plans to incorporate more teachings of self-help, finance and meditation. Regular meditation is very beneficial to her progress as she forges a new life. Morning rituals and positive incantations are other practices Michele embraces; they are very restorative in daily life.

As an avid hiker, Michele and fellow club members often hike the picturesque Jersey Pine Barrens. She is a history buff, voracious reader, baseball fanatic and a foodie. She also proudly supports Trout Unlimited-a national non-profit organization dedicated to conserving, protecting and restoring North America's Coldwater fisheries and their watersheds.

Michele currently resides forty minutes from Atlantic City and the Jersey Shore. She makes her home with a Blue Russian rescue cat named Jersey, though she isn't exactly sure who rescued who.

Michele really enjoys publishing books that can make a difference in people's lives. If you have any suggestions or would like to have a specific topic covered in a future book, please send an email to michelegilbertbooks@gmail.com and we will get back to you.

Thanks for reading!

www.ingramcontent.com/pod-product-compliance
Lightning Source LLC
Chambersburg PA
CBHW040842180526
45159CB00001B/286